Nourish and Flourish: 3-month easy weight loss

"A 3-month sustainable approach for men and women"

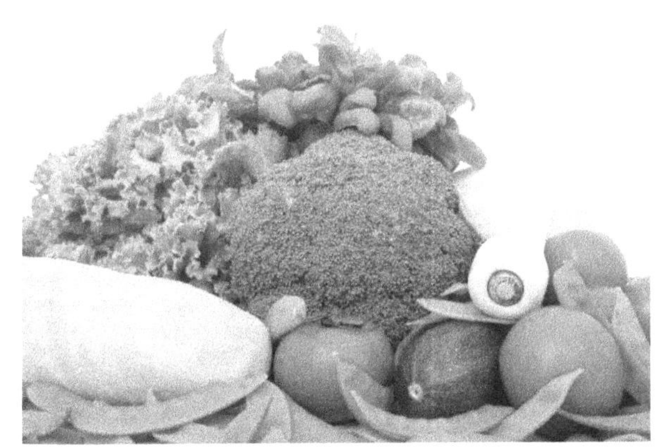

DA SILVA

Copyright © 2024 by DA SILVA

All rights reserved.

No part of this book may be reproduced, stored in a retrieval system, or transmitted in any form or by any means, electronic, mechanical, photocopying, recording, or otherwise, without the prior written permission of the author.

Table of Contents

Introduction

Oh, dear friend, i write this book with tears in my eyes, thinking about the long, hard journey that brought me to this place of peace and freedom. For 5 years, I struggled with my weight, feeling like a prisoner in my own body. I tried every fad diet, every exercise program, every quick fix, but nothing seemed to work for long. I forgot the feeling of confidence as I always felt isolated especially from this present day society.

But here's the thing; I didn't have anyone to guide me, anyone to show me the way. I had to figure it out on my own, through trial and error, and it took me 5 years to finally achieve the effortless weight loss I'd always dreamed of.

But you don't have to go that far, dear friend. I want to spare you the struggle, the pain, and the frustration. I will share with you the **secrets** I've learned, the **strategies** that finally worked for me, so that you can achieve in **3 months** what took me 5 years.

That's why I'm writing this book. I'm sharing my story with you because I know that you don't have to suffer like I did. I know that you can find freedom, peace, and self-love in just a few short months. I'll guide you all the way.

Chapter 1: Healthy Eating Habits (Days 1-30)

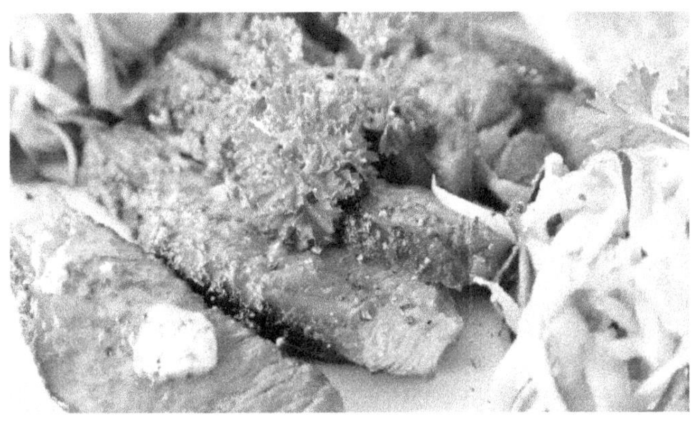

The foundation of effortless weight loss begins with healthy eating habits. In this chapter, we'll explore the power of whole foods, portion control, and mindful eating. You'll learn how to nourish your body with the right foods, in the right amounts, to support your weight loss journey.

By adopting these healthy eating habits, you'll be amazed at how easily you can shed those extra pounds and maintain a healthy weight for the long-term. Let's dive in and start building the foundation for your weight loss success.

Focus on whole foods:

Whole foods are the key to unlocking effortless weight loss. By focusing on whole, unprocessed foods like vegetables, fruits, whole grains, lean proteins, and healthy fats, you'll be giving your body the nutrients it needs to function at its best.

Say goodbye to fad diets and processed snacks, and hello to a **balanced** and **sustainable** approach to weight loss. Let's explore the benefits of whole foods and how the foundation your weight loss journey.

Fruits

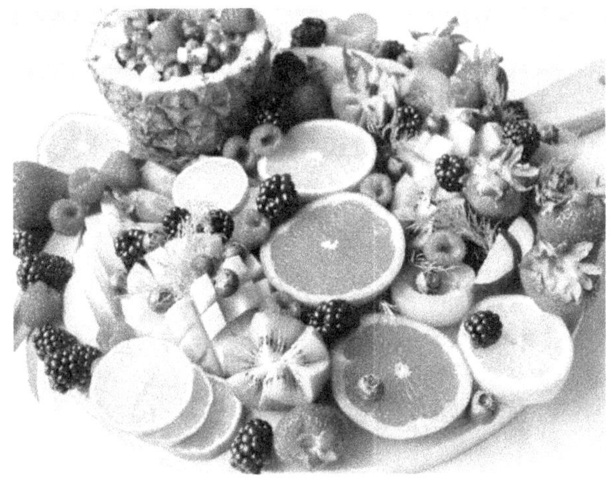

Fruits are a vital part of a whole food diet, and they offer numerous benefits for adults in their 30s to 60s. As we age, our bodies undergo a range of changes that can affect our weight, energy levels, and overall health. Fruits are rich in antioxidants, fiber, and essential vitamins and minerals that can help:

- **Boost metabolism and support weight loss**

Fruits like **apples**, **berries**, and **citrus fruits** are high in fiber, which helps speed up digestion and keep us feeling fuller for longer. This can lead to a natural boost in metabolism, supporting weight loss and weight management, especially as we age and the speed of metabolism determines how fast our bodies burn calories.

- **Support healthy digestion and prevent constipation**

Fruits like **bananas**, **apricots**, and **prunes** are rich in dietary fiber, which can help regulate bowel movements and prevent constipation. This is especially important in our 30s to 60s, as our digestive systems may slow down with age.

- **Reduce inflammation and improve overall health**

Fruits like **pomegranates**, **grapes**, and **berries** are packed with antioxidants and polyphenols, which can help reduce inflammation and oxidative stress in our bodies. This can lead to improved overall health and reduced risk of chronic diseases, such as heart disease, diabetes, and certain cancers.

- **Provide essential vitamins and minerals**

Fruits like **papaya**, **cantaloupe**, and **strawberries** are rich in vitamins A and C, potassium, and other essential nutrients that support healthy skin, hair, and nail growth. This can help combat signs of aging, such as wrinkles, dry skin, and brittle hair and nails.

Vegetables

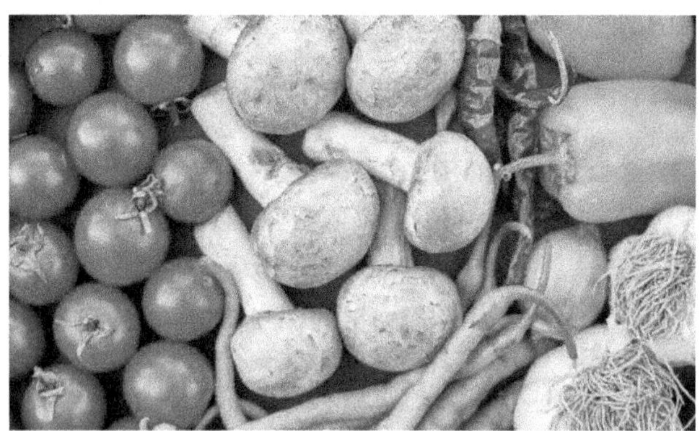

Vegetables are a secret weapon for weight loss and overall health in our 30s to 60s. They're low in calories, rich in fiber, and packed with water content, making them a filling and satisfying addition to our diets.

Plus, they're incredibly versatile. Enjoy them as a snack, side dish, or added to your favorite recipes to boost nutrition and flavor!

Here are a few examples of vegetables your can incorporate in your own meals:

- Adding carrots and onions to soups and stews.
- Baking or boiling potatoes as a side dish.
- Using canned tomatoes in sauces and soups.

- Adding frozen peas to rice dishes or omelets.
- Using canned beans in salads, soups, or as a protein source.
- Making coleslaw with cabbage and carrots.
- Snacking on celery sticks with hummus.
- Adding frozen spinach to smoothies or omelets.
- Steaming green beans as a side dish.

Whole grains

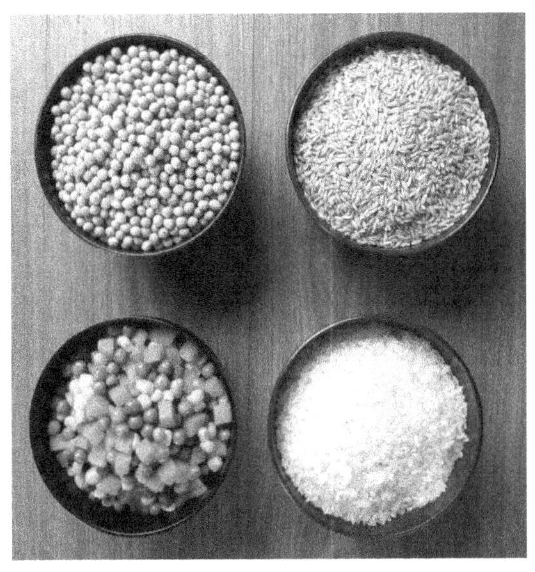

Whole grains are a nutritional powerhouse, supporting weight loss and overall health in our 30s to 60s. They are packed with nutrients including fiber, vitamins and minerals that can:

- Lower cholesterol and blood pressure
- Regulate blood sugar levels
- Keep you feeling fuller longer
- Support healthy digestion

Incorporate whole grains like **brown rice**, **quinoa**, **whole wheat bread**, and **whole grain pasta** into your meals to reap the benefits.

Lean meats

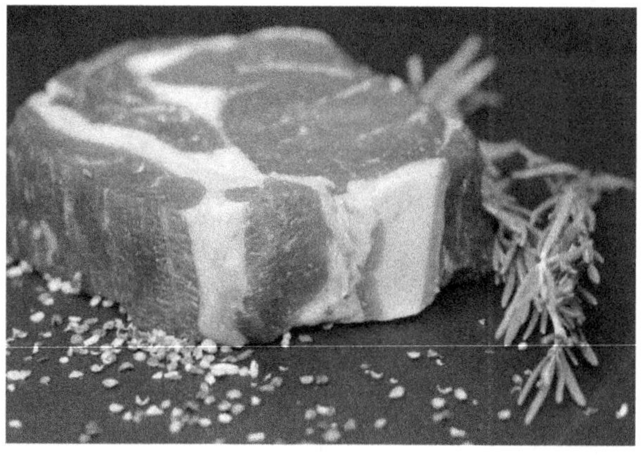

Lean meats are an essential protein source, supporting weight loss and overall health in our 30s to 60s. They're rich in protein, vitamins, and minerals that can help:

- Build and repair muscles

- Keep you feeling fuller longer

- Support healthy bones

- Boost metabolism

Choose lean meats like **chicken**, **turkey**, **fish**, and **lean beef** to reap the benefits.

Low-fat dairy

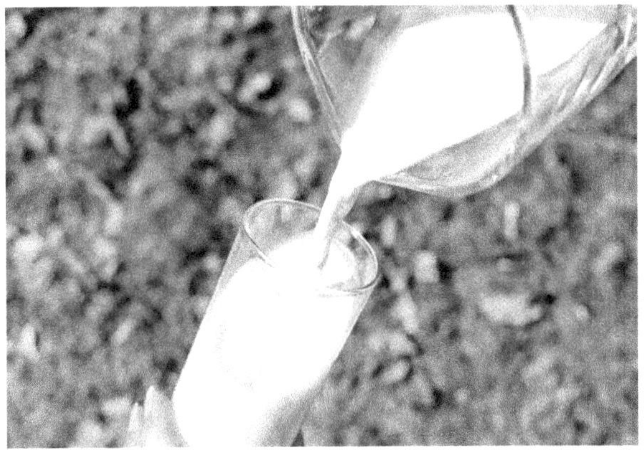

Low-fat dairy is a nutritious addition to a weight loss diet, supporting overall health in our 30s to 60s. It's rich in:

- Calcium for strong bones
- Protein for muscle health
- Potassium for healthy blood pressure
- Probiotics for gut health

Choose low-fat or fat-free options like **milk**, **yogurt**, and **cheese** to reap the benefits while keeping calories in check.

Here are some meal plan suggestions incorporating fruits, vegetables, whole grains, lean meats, and low-fat dairy I still use almost everyday:

For Breakfast;

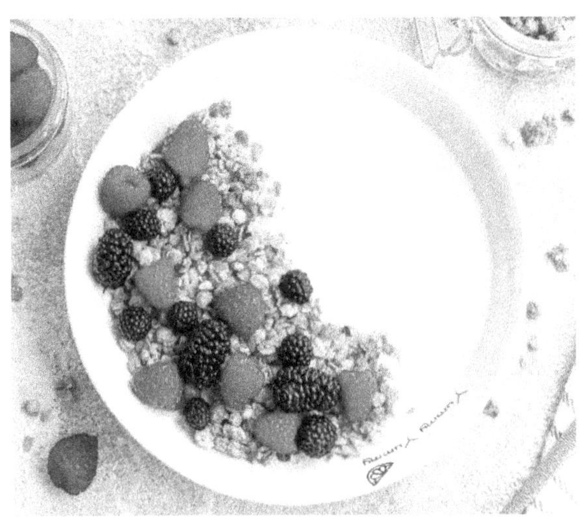

- **Fruit:** Berries (blueberries, strawberries, raspberries)
- **Meal:** Greek Yogurt Parfait with Granola and Berries

Recipe:

- **1 cup** low-fat Greek yogurt
- **2 tbsp** granola
- **1 cup** mixed berries
- **1 slice** whole grain toast

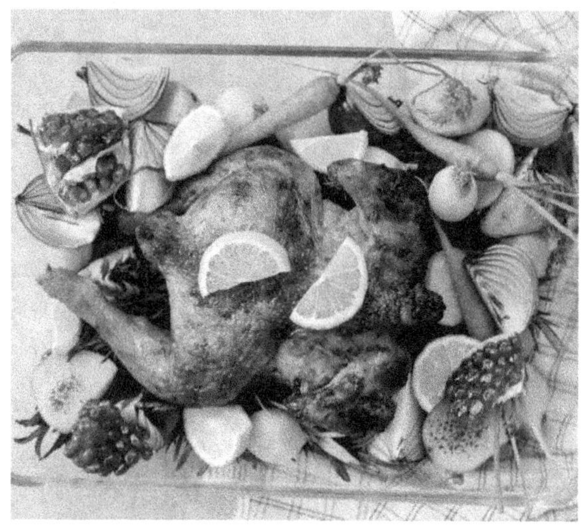

Fruit: Apple/Orange

Meal: Grilled Chicken with Veggie Wrap with orange Slices and onions.

Recipe:

- **1 whole** wheat tortilla
- **4 oz** grilled chicken breast
- **1 cup** mixed greens

- **1/2 cup** sliced cucumber

- **1/2 cup** sliced bell peppers

- **1/2 orange**, sliced

- **1/2 onions**, sliced

For Dinner;

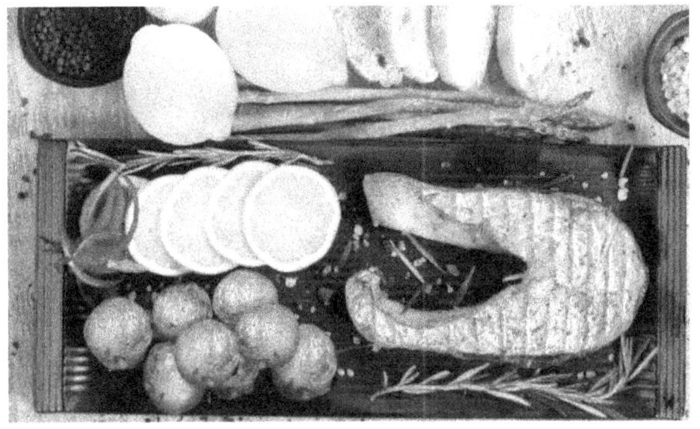

- **Fruit:** Orange

- **Meal:** Baked Salmon with Roasted Veggies and Orange Slices

Recipe:

- **6 oz** salmon fillet

- **1 cup** mixed veggies (broccoli, carrots, sweet potatoes)
- **1 orange**, sliced
- **1 cup** cooked quinoa

For a Snack;

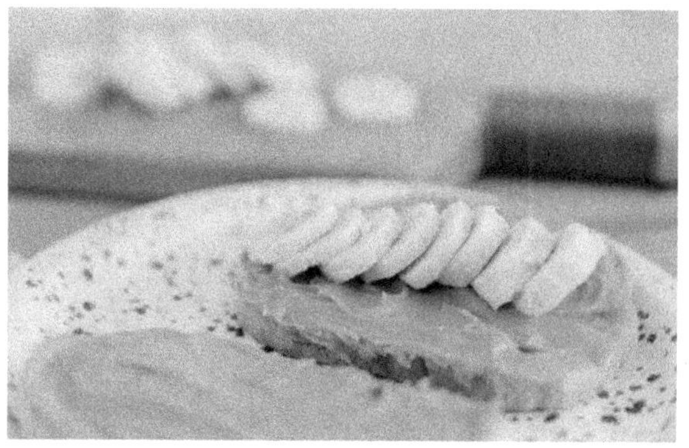

- **Fruit:** Banana
- **Meal:** Banana and Peanut Butter sandwich with Low-Fat Milk

Recipe:

- **1 banana**

- **2 tbsp** peanut butter
- **1 cup** low-fat milk
- **1/2 cup** Greek yogurt
- **Two slices** of bread.

Allowance for occasional sugary snacks (1–2 times a week)

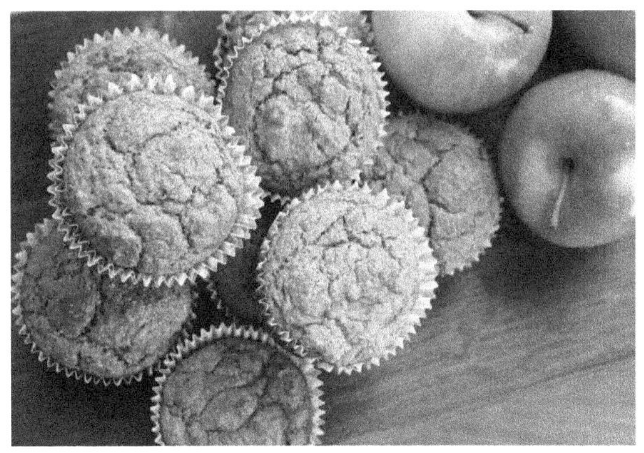

Embarking on a weight loss journey doesn't have to mean completely depriving yourself of sweet treats. In fact, allowing for occasional sugary snacks can actually help you stay on track and achieve your goals.

By incorporating small indulgences into your diet, you'll be more likely to stick to your healthy eating plan and avoid feelings of restriction and deprivation.

It allows for a sustainable and balanced approach to dieting. By permitting yourself the occasional sugary snack, you'll experience several benefits like:
- Reduced feelings of deprivation, which can lead to overindulgence.
- Increased flexibility and adaptability in social situations
- Improved mental health and stress reduction related to restrictive eating

- Enhanced overall enjoyment of healthy foods, without feeling restricted
- A more maintainable and long-term approach to weight loss, rather than a quick fix

Here are some tips and strategies for incorporating sugary snacks into your diet in a way that supports your weight loss goals:

1. **Set a weekly limit:** Allow yourself 1-2 sugary snacks per week, and stick to it.

2. **Choose smaller portions:** Opt for smaller servings or "mini" versions of your favorite treats.

3. **Balance with healthy choices:** Make sure your daily diet is filled with nutrient-dense foods, and use sugary snacks as an occasional treat.

4. **Plan ahead:** Schedule your sugary snacks in advance, so you don't impulsively reach for them.

5. **Savor and enjoy:** Eat your sugary snacks slowly and mindfully, savoring every bite.

6. **Don't keep them at home:** Avoid storing sugary snacks in your house to reduce temptation.

7. **Find healthier alternatives:** Discover lower-calorie versions of your favorite treats or try new healthier options.

8. **Be mindful of hidden sugars:** Pay attention to added sugars in foods like yogurt, granola, and sauces.

9. **Use the 10-minute rule:** Wait 10 minutes before indulging in a sugary snack to assess if you're truly hungry.

10. **Stay hydrated:** Sometimes thirst can masquerade as hunger, so drink water before reaching for a snack.

Remember, **moderation is key.** By following these tips, you can enjoy sugary snacks while still achieving your weight loss goals. Also don't forget to practice walking, jogging, and other exercises to help burn out calories and build muscle.

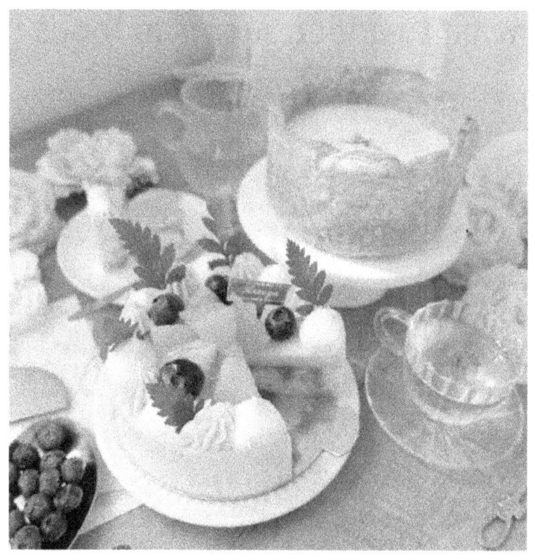

Chapter 2: Gender-specific nutrition considerations:

When it comes to weight loss, a one-size-fits-all approach often falls short. Men and women have distinct physiological differences that impact their nutritional needs and weight loss strategies. Understanding these gender-specific considerations can be the key to unlocking successful weight loss.

In this chapter, we'll explore the unique nutritional needs of men and women, and provide tailored guidance on how to fuel your body for optimal weight loss results.

Whether you're a man looking to **boost testosterone levels** or a woman seeking to **balance hormones**, this chapter will provide the insights you need to achieve your weight loss goals.

Men: protein-rich foods for muscle mass, healthy fats for testosterone

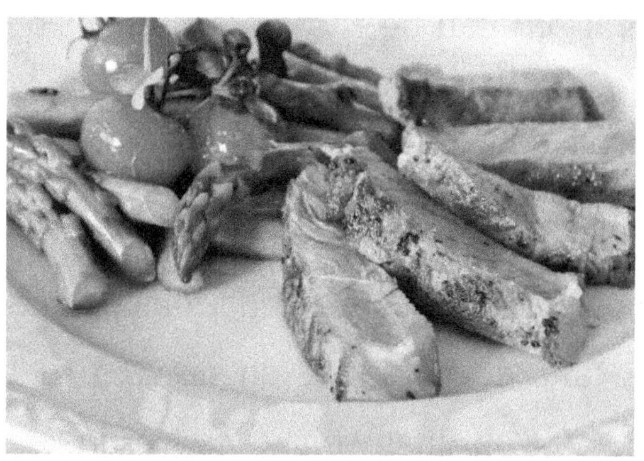

When it comes to **optimizing testosterone levels** and **building muscle mass**, men require a specific balance of nutrients. Here are the key considerations:

1. **Protein:** Aim for 1.**6-2.2 grams** of protein per kilogram of body weight from sources like **lean meats, fish, eggs, dairy,** and plant-based options like **legumes** and **nuts.**

2. **Healthy Fats:** Include sources like **avocados, nuts,** and **olive oil** in your diet to support hormone production and overall health.

3. **Vitamin D:** Ensure adequate vitamin D levels through sun exposure, supplements, or fortified foods like **milk** and **cereal.**

4. **Zinc:** Include zinc-rich foods like **oysters**, **beef**, **chicken**, and fortified cereals to support testosterone production.

5. **Magnesium:** Aim for **400-420 mg** of magnesium per day from sources like dark **leafy greens**, **nuts**, and **whole grains**.

6. **Creatine:** Consider supplementing with creatine to increase muscle strength and endurance.

7. **Beta-Alanine:** Include beta-alanine-rich foods like **meat**, **fish**, and **poultry** to support muscle carnosine production.

8. **Branched-Chain Amino Acids (BCAAs):** Consider supplementing with BCAAs to support muscle growth and recovery.

By focusing on these nutritional needs, men can support optimal testosterone levels, muscle growth, and overall health. Remember to always consult with a healthcare professional or registered dietitian before starting any new supplements.

Women: iron-rich foods, calcium-rich foods, and healthy fats for hormone balance

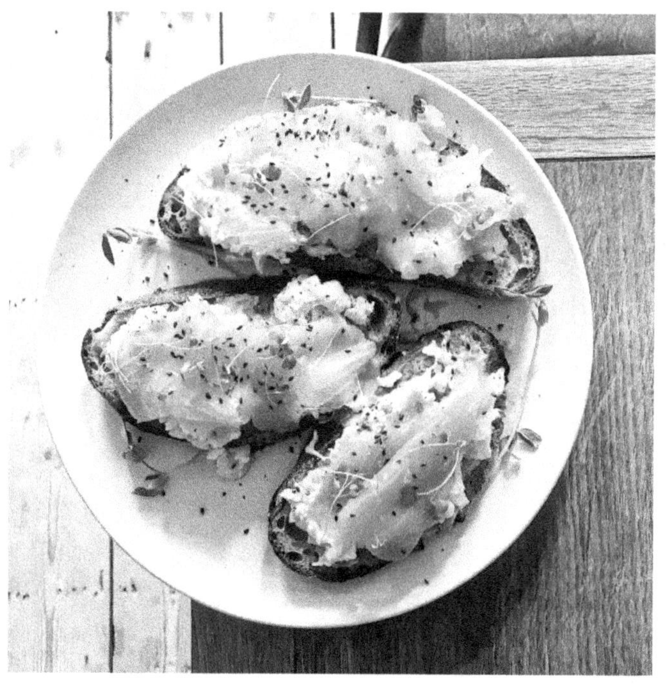

A balanced diet is essential for women seeking to balance their hormones. Here are some key nutritional needs:

1. **Omega-3 Fatty Acids:** Supports hormone production and reduces inflammation. Find them in **fatty fish**, **flaxseeds**, and **walnuts**.

2. **Probiotics:** Maintains gut health, crucial for hormone regulation. Enjoy probiotic-rich foods like **yogurt**, **kefir**, and **fermented vegetables**.

3. **Vitamin D:** Essential for hormone balance and overall health. Get it through sunlight, supplements, or vitamin D-rich foods like **fatty fish** and **egg yolks**.

4. **Magnesium**: Helps regulate hormones and alleviates symptoms like cramps and mood swings. Include magnesium-rich foods like **dark leafy greens, nuts**, and **seeds in your diet.**

5. **Antioxidants:** Reduces oxidative stress and inflammation, supporting hormone balance. Find antioxidants in **berries, leafy greens**, and other fruits and vegetables.

6. **Whole Grains:** Provides fiber, vitamins, and minerals essential for hormone regulation. Choose whole grains like **brown rice, quinoa**, and **whole-wheat bread.**

7. **Lean Protein:** Supports hormone production and overall health. Include lean protein sources like **poultry, fish, beans,** and **lentils** in your diet.

8. **Healthy Fats:** Essential for hormone production and balance. Nourish your body with healthy fats from **avocados, olive oil,** and **nuts.**

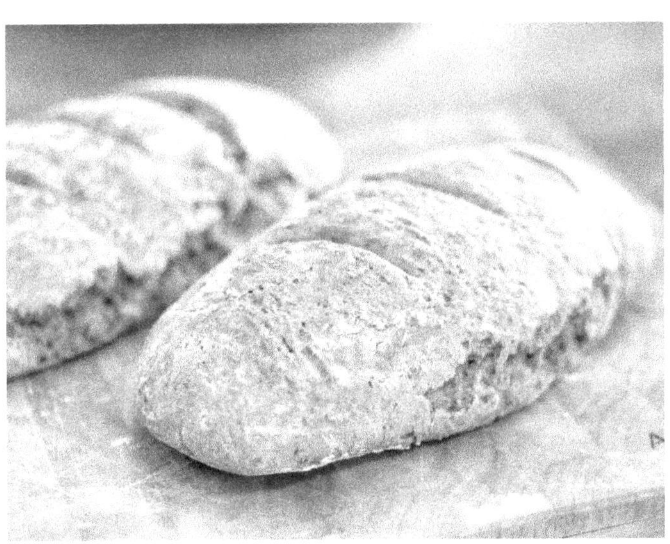

By incorporating these nutritional powerhouses into your diet, you'll be supporting your hormonal balance and overall well-being.

Chapter 3: Meal Timing

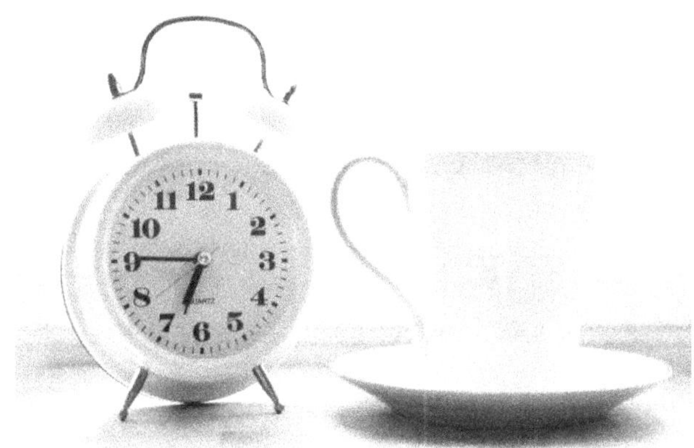

When it comes to weight loss, it's not just about **what you eat**, but also **when you eat**. Strategic meal timing and snacking can boost your metabolism, control hunger, and support sustainable weight loss.

Eat 3 main meals and 2 snacks daily

As we age, our metabolism slows, and our bodies require more support to maintain weight loss. Eating 3 main meals and 2 snacks daily can help:

1. **Prevents Extreme Hunger:** Spacing out meals and snacks throughout the day prevents extreme hunger, reducing the likelihood of overeating.

2. **Controls Portion Sizes:** Eating smaller, frequent meals helps regulate portion sizes, making it easier to stick to appropriate serving sizes.

3. **Reduces Mindless Snacking:** Including 2 snacks in your daily routine reduces the need for mindless snacking, which can lead to consuming excess calories.

4. **Stabilizes Blood Sugar:** Eating regular meals and snacks helps maintain stable blood sugar levels, reducing cravings for unhealthy foods and overeating.

5. **Supports Healthy Digestion:** A balanced eating pattern promotes healthy digestion, reducing symptoms like bloating and discomfort that may lead to overeating.

By incorporating this eating pattern, you'll be better equipped to manage hunger, control portion sizes, and develop a healthier relationship with food, ultimately reducing the likelihood of overeating and supporting sustainable weight loss.

Optimal timing for meals and snacks

This is a very important factor that can cause health problems if overlooked.

Optimal Timing for Meals:

Here's a suggested meal timing plan I use to help avoid indigestion and overweight:

Breakfast (7:00-8:00 am)

- Kick Starts your metabolism
- Helps regulate blood sugar levels

Mid-Morning Snack (10:00-11:00 am)

- Prevents extreme hunger
- Supports energy levels

Lunch (12:00-1:00 pm)

- Provides energy for the day

- Helps maintain focus and productivity

Mid-Afternoon Snack (3:00-4:00 pm)

- Boosts energy levels
- Reduces cravings for unhealthy snacks

Dinner (6:00-7:00 pm)

- Supports relaxation and digestion
- Helps regulate blood sugar levels

Evening Snack (Optional) (8:00-9:00 pm)

- **Only if necessary,** to prevent extreme hunger before bed
- **Choose a light,** balanced snack

This timing plan allows for:

- 3 main meals
- 2 snacks
- Adequate time for digestion

- Reduced likelihood of overeating
- Boosted metabolism and energy levels

"Remember, eating a late night meal (after 7pm) is not always healthy if at all it ever is". This plays a huge role on weight gain especially for us middle-aged adults because of the following reasons:

1. **Slower Digestion:** As we age, our digestive system slows down, making it more challenging to digest food efficiently, especially in the evening.

2. **Reduced Stomach Acid:** Stomach acid production decreases with age, making it harder to break down food, leading to indigestion and bloating.

3. **Hormonal Changes:** Hormonal fluctuations during aging can affect

digestion, leading to slower gut motility and increased bloating.

4. **Relaxed Lower Esophageal Sphincter:** The muscle that separates the esophagus and stomach relaxes with age, allowing stomach acid to flow back up, causing discomfort and bloating.

5. **Poor Sleep:** Eating close to bedtime can disrupt sleep quality, further exacerbating digestive issues.

To minimize bloating and indigestion, consider finishing your main meal by 7pm and opting for a light, balanced snack if needed later in the evening. This allows for:

- Adequate digestion time
- Reduced discomfort during sleep
- Improved overall digestive health

Remember also, that everyone's body is different, so it's essential to listen to your body and adjust your eating schedule accordingly.

In summary, for the first month of your weight loss journey, you will need to understand:

- How your body works
- What type of meals it requires.
- When it requires each meal.
- How much of it (meal) your body requires.

This can especially help prevent **pointless starvation** or **overeating**.

Chapter 4: Portion Control and Mindful Eating (Days 31-60)

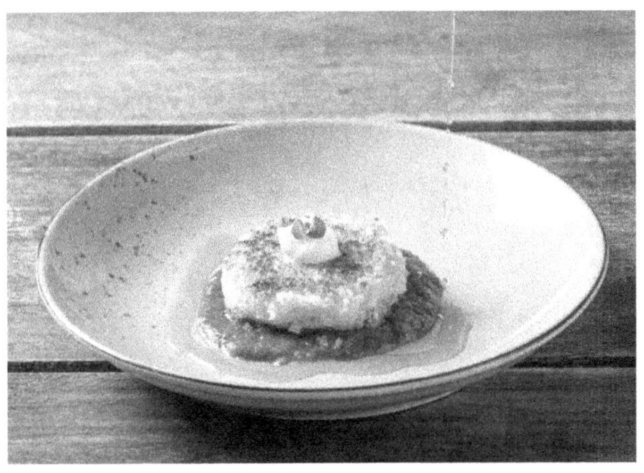

For the second month, you will learn to take control of your weight loss journey by mastering the part of portion control and mindful eating.

As a bonus tip, I'll guide you through the next 30 days of your transformation, helping you develop healthy habits that will stick. You'll learn how to:

- Eat appropriate serving sizes
- Savor each bite
- Recognize hunger and fullness cues
- Avoid emotional eating
- Develop a healthier relationship with food

Portion control Time table

By practicing portion control and mindful eating, you'll experience sustainable weight loss, improved digestion, and a renewed sense of well-being. Try out the following for the second month of your weight loss journey;

DAY	HABIT	ACTION
1 - 5	Eat **3** main meals and **2** snacks.	Plan meals
	Drink **8** glasses of water.	Keep a water bottle with you
	Morning stretches	Find a quiet place for stretching
6 - 15	Food Diary	Write down everything you eat and drink. Include **portion sizes**, and **hunger levels**
	Replace sugary	Try unsweetened

	drinks	tea or coffee, infused water with fruits or herbs
	10 minute walks	Find a nearby park or street
16 - 20	Portion Control	Make use of **food scale** or **measuring cup**, eat slowly and mindfully
	Mindful eating	Savor each bite while paying attention to flavour and texture.
	Strength Training	Find a workout routine online; Start lightly and gradually increase

21 - 25	Identify emotional eating triggers along the way	Reflect on **when** and **why** you eat; Find healthy alternatives
	Healthy Snacks	Try **fruits**, **nuts**, or **carrot sticks with hummus**
	Deep breathing exercises	Find a quiet place, focus on slow deep breaths
26 - 30	Meal preparation and planning	Make a meal plan and prepare ingredients in advance
	Cardio exercises	Find a workout routine online, gradually start

		and increase
	Progress reflection	Review food diaries and progress photos. Celebrate success with new goals

Avoid eating in front of screens or while stressed

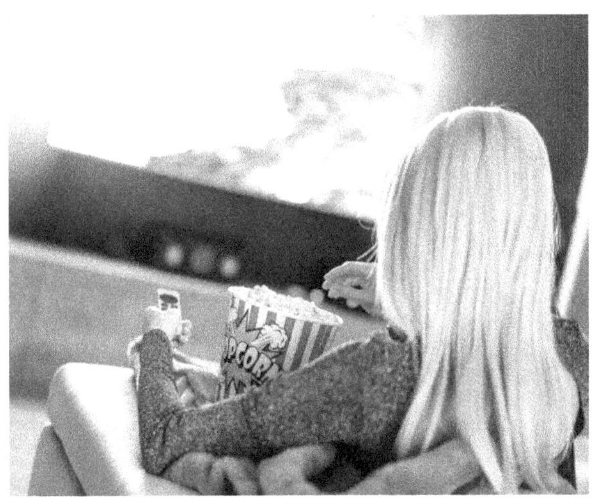

Try to avoid eating in front of screens or while stressed as this could contribute hugely on weight gain. Here's why:

Eating in front of screens (TV, phone, computer, etc.) can lead to:
- Mindless snacking
- Overeating

- Poor food choices
- Reduced awareness of hunger and fullness cues

Eating while stressed can lead to:
- Emotional eating
- Comfort food cravings
- Overeating or undereating
- Disrupted digestion and nutrient absorption

Remember, eating is not just about fueling your body; it's also about nourishing your mind and spirit. By being present and mindful during meals, you can cultivate a more balanced and joyful relationship with food.

Chapter 5: Exercise (Days 1-60)

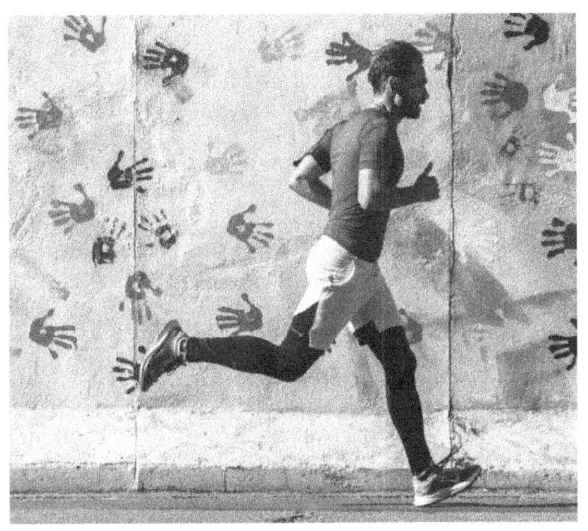

From our table above, you can notice that exercise training starts from the **16th - 30th day**. But that doesn't mean you only need to exercise in the second month; The exercise starts from the second month.

Let's dive into the exercise component of the transformation guide.

Exercise Days (Days 16–30)

Aim for at least 30 minutes of moderate-intensity exercise per day, divided into:

- Morning (15-20 minutes)
- Afternoon (10-15 minutes, optional)
- Night (10-15 minutes)

Morning Exercises (Men and Women)

1. Brisk Walking

2. Jumping Jacks

3. Bodyweight Squats

4. Push-ups

5. Plank Hold

6. Yoga (sun salutations, warrior poses, etc.)

Afternoon Exercises (Optional, Men and Women)

1. Short Walk or Jog

2. Stair Climbing

3. Bodyweight Lunges

4. Dumbbell Rows (using water bottles or cans)

5. Shoulder Press (using light weights or resistance bands)

Night Exercises (Men and Women)

1. Gentle Stretching

2. Yoga (gentle flows, downward-facing dog, etc.)

3. Bodyweight Leg Raises

4. Wall Sit

5. Light Cardio (jogging in place, jumping jacks, etc.)

Additional Tips

- Warm up with 5-10 minutes of light cardio before each exercise session
- Cool down with 5-10 minutes of stretching after each session
- Listen to your body and rest when needed
- Increase intensity and duration as you progress
- Consult a healthcare professional before starting any new exercise program

Remember, **"Consistency and Progress are key"**. Start with manageable exercises and gradually increase intensity and duration as you become more comfortable. Make exercise a habit, and you'll be on your way to a healthier, happier you!

Chapter 6: Lifestyle Changes (Days 1-90)

We'll now look into your sleep and stress management. Obviously a task for change can be stressful, but there are many ways to counter stress.

Stress Management

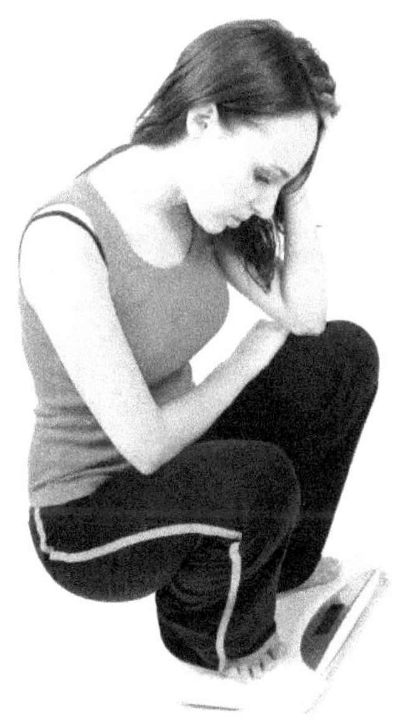

While following the weight loss guide, it's essential to manage stress levels to avoid emotional eating and promote overall well-being. Try any of these stress-reducing techniques:

1. **Deep Breathing Exercises:** Take 5-10 minutes to focus on slow, deep breaths, inhaling through your nose and exhaling through your mouth.

2. **Mindfulness Meditation:** Use apps like Headspace or Calm to guide you through meditation sessions.

3. **Yoga:** Practice gentle yoga stretches to relax your mind and body.

4. **Journaling:** Write down your thoughts and feelings to process and release emotions. This one especially works for me as it also helps me keep track of my progress.

5. **Short Walks:** Take a 10-minute walk outside to clear your mind and reduce stress. Observe your surroundings and make future plans.

Sleep Management

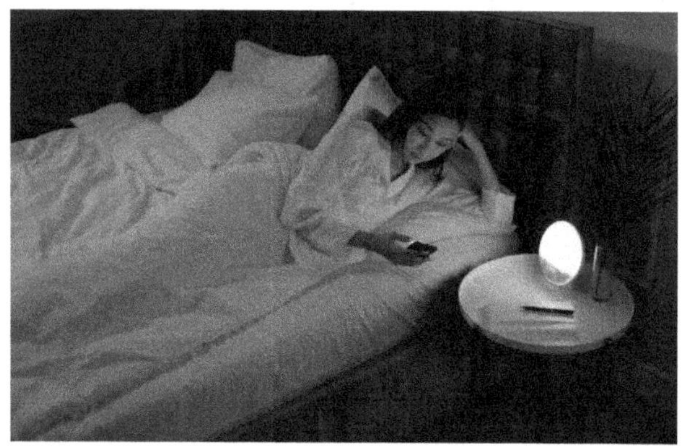

Aim for **7-9 hours of sleep** each night to support weight loss and overall health. Try these sleep-enhancing tips:

1. **Establish a Bedtime Routine:** Wind down with a warm bath, reading, or relaxation techniques.

2. **Stick to a Sleep Schedule:** Go to bed and wake up at the same time every day, including weekends.

3. **Create a Sleep-Conducive Environment:** Make your bedroom dark, quiet, and cool.

4. **Avoid Screens Before Bed:** Try to avoid screens for at least an hour before bedtime.

5. **Limit Caffeine and Alcohol:** Avoid consuming these substances in the hours leading up to bedtime.

Additional Tips

- Prioritize self-care and make time for activities that bring you joy and relaxation.
- Learn to say "no" to commitments that may interfere with your sleep and stress management goals.

- Consider seeking support from friends, family, or a therapist if you're struggling with stress or sleep.

Remember, managing stress and sleep is crucial for overall health and weight loss. By incorporating these techniques into your daily routine, you'll be better equipped to handle stress and get the restful sleep your body needs.

Conclusion: Progress Tracking and Motivation

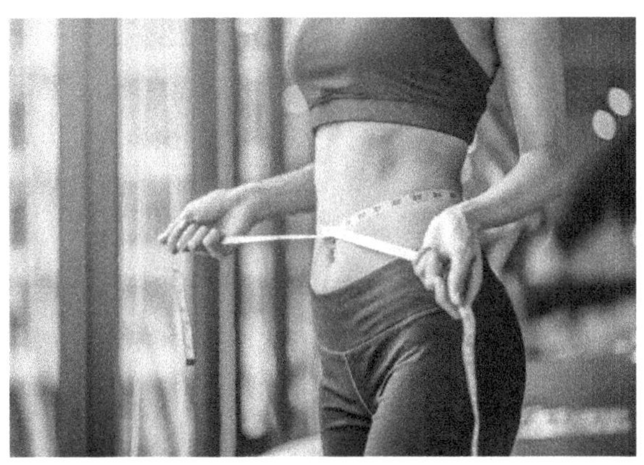

Congratulations on reaching the final stretch of your 90-day transformation journey. You've worked hard to develop healthy habits, and it's essential to track your progress and stay motivated to maintain your success.

Progress Tracking:

1. **Weight and Measurements:** Take progress photos and track your weight, measurements, and body fat percentage.

2. **Food Diary:** Continue logging your food intake to monitor your eating habits.

3. **Workout Log:** Record your exercises, sets, reps, and weight lifted.

4. **Mood and Energy:** Track your mood, energy levels, and overall well-being.

Motivation:

1. **Celebrate Milestones:** Reward yourself for reaching goals and milestones.
2. **Accountability Partner:** Share your progress with a friend or family member for support.
3. **Inspiration:** Follow fitness influencers, read motivational stories, or watch workout videos.
4. **Self-Care:** Prioritize rest, relaxation, and self-care activities.

Remember, this journey is just the beginning. Stay committed, and you'll continue to see amazing results.

Let's meet again in 90 days to celebrate your continued success and set new goals. Keep shining, and remember: health is wealth!

Until we meet again, stay healthy, happy, and motivated!

Your Health and Wellness Coach,
DA SILVA

www.ingramcontent.com/pod-product-compliance
Lightning Source LLC
Chambersburg PA
CBHW070803250726

48662CB00004B/1952